KNOWLEDGE GUIDE TO ROTATOR CUFF TEARS

Essential Manual To Prevention, Diagnosis, Treatment, And Rehabilitation For Shoulder Pain Relief

DR. AARON BRANUM

Copyright © 2024 BY DR. AARON BRANUM

All rights reserved. Except for brief quotations embodied in critical reviews and certain other noncommercial uses permitted by copyright law, no part of this publication may be reproduced, distributed, or transmitted in any form or by any means, Including photocopying, recording, or other electronic or mechanical methods, without the prior written permission of the publisher.

Disclaimer:

The data in this book, is solely meant to be informative and instructional.

This book is not intended to replace expert medical advice, diagnosis, or care. No medical, health, or other professional services are offered by the author, publisher, or any affiliated parties

Individual outcomes may differ in the practice of these therapies, which entail a variety of approaches and methodologies.

A one-on-one session with a trained or certified healthcare professional is still preferable. It is best to consult a trained healthcare provider before making any decisions regarding your health.

The author of this book is not affiliated with any specific website, product, or organization related to any of these therapies.

All reasonable measures have been taken by the author and publisher to guarantee the authenticity and dependability of the material contained in this book

Contents

CHAPTER ONE 13
DESCRIPTION OF THE SHOULDER 13
The Anatomy And Physiology Of The Shoulder Joint 13

The Rotator Cuff Muscles' Function 14

The Value Of Stability In The Shoulders ...15

Recognizing The Range Of Motion In The Shoulders 16

Typical Injuries To The Shoulders............18

CHAPTER TWO 21
ROTATOR CUFF TEARS: TYPES...................21
Tears Of Partial Vs. Full Thickness 21

Acute versus Prolonged Tears 22

Where And How Much Weeping There Is ..23

Factors Affecting The Formation Of Tears .25

Diagnostic Imaging Methods...................26

CHAPTER THREE 29
RISK ELEMENTS AND ACTIONS 29
Increasing Age And Degenerative Modifications 29

Overindulgence And Repetitive Motions....30

　　Shoulder Accidents And Traumas 31

　　Techniques For Preventing Injuries..........32

　　Lifestyle Changes For The Health Of The
　　Shoulders 33

CHAPTER FOUR...35

　DIAGNOSIS AND ASSESSMENT..................35

　　Medical Professionals' Clinical Evaluation ..35

　　Imaging Studies: Mris, Ultrasounds, And X-
　　Rays 36

　　Methods Of Physical Examination 38

　　Differential Shoulder Pain Diagnosis.........39

　　The Value Of Extensive Analysis..............41

CHAPTER FIVE 43

　SELECTIVE NON-SURGICAL ROTATOR CUFF
　TEAR TREATMENT OPTIONS......................43

　　Elevation, Compression, Ice, Rest (RICE) .43

　　Rehabilitation And Physical Therapy.........44

　　Pain And Inflammation Medicines 46

　　Injections Of Corticosteroids...................47

Treatment With Platelet-Rich Plasma (PRP) 49

CHAPTER SIX 51

  SURGICAL ASSISTANCE 51

    Reasons To Operate 51

    Surgical Procedure Types 52

    Open Vs Arthroscopic Surgery 54

    Recovery After Surgery 55

    Possible Dangers And Issues 58

CHAPTER SEVEN 61

  CARE AFTER POSTOPERATION AND REHABILITATION 61

    Postoperative Rehabilitation's Significance 61

    Exercises For Range Of Motion 62

    Programs For Strengthening And Conditioning 63

    Returning To Activities Gradually 64

    Keeping An Eye Out For Complications Or Recurrence 65

CHAPTER EIGHT 67

CHANGES IN LIFESTYLE AND LONG-TERM MANAGEMENT 67
   Ergonomic Adjustments To Stop Recurrence 67
   Nutrition And Hydration's Role 68
   The Value Of Frequent Exercise............... 69
   Stress Reduction And Mental Health 70
   Long-Term Care Follow-Up With Medical Professionals 71

CHAPTER NINE.. 73
   COMMON QUESTIONS AND ANSWERS 73
      Can Tears In The Rotator Cuff Heal On Their Own? 73
      What Are Surgical Intervention Success Rates?... 74
      How Much Time Does Recovery Take?...... 75
      After Treatment, Will My Whole Range Of Motion Return? 76
      How Can I Avoid Shoulder Injuries In The Future?... 77

CONCERNING THIS BOOK

If one wants a thorough understanding of rotator cuff injuries, the book "Knowledge Guide to Rotator Cuff Tears" is an essential reference. Every facet of rotator cuff tears is thoroughly covered in this book, from the fundamentals of shoulder anatomy to the intricacies of long-term therapy and postoperative care. Through an exploration of the complexities surrounding the shoulder joint and the essential function of the rotator cuff muscles, readers acquire a fundamental understanding that emphasizes the significance of shoulder stability and mobility. The thorough examination of frequent shoulder injuries and the many kinds of rotator cuff tears improves readers' diagnostic acumen by teaching them to distinguish between partial and full-thickness rips, as well as between acute and chronic disorders.

For both prevention and therapy, it is essential to comprehend the various causes of rotator cuff tears, including age-related degenerative changes, overuse, repetitive movements, and trauma. In addition to explaining these risk factors, this guide offers doable methods for preventing injuries and making lifestyle changes that will preserve shoulder health. The focus on early detection and the thorough review of diagnostic imaging methods, including MRIs, ultrasounds, and X-rays, emphasize how important a precise diagnosis is to efficient treatment planning.

The extensive coverage of both surgical and non-surgical treatment methods in the book guarantees that readers have a complete understanding of the range of care alternatives.

Clear explanations of non-surgical treatments like physical therapy, RICE, drugs, and cutting-edge therapies like PRP therapy are provided, providing good substitutes for individuals who would prefer not to have surgery. The book describes a variety of surgical treatments, such as open and arthroscopic surgery, and the dangers and recovery processes involved for individuals who need them.

The need for a planned rehabilitation program to regain range of motion, strength, and function is highlighted by the substantial attention that is paid to postoperative care and rehabilitation. The handbook also covers long-term management techniques to stop recurrence and enhance general well-being, like dietary modifications, regular exercise, ergonomic adjustments, and mental health assistance. This book is a vital resource for patients, healthcare professionals, and anybody else interested in preserving the best possible shoulder health because it includes common concerns and FAQs that offer useful solutions to often-asked issues.

All things considered, "Knowledge Guide to Rotator Cuff Tears" is an authoritative resource that blends medical knowledge with helpful guidance, guaranteeing that readers have the information and resources necessary to successfully negotiate the complexity of rotator cuff injuries and their care.

CHAPTER ONE

DESCRIPTION OF THE SHOULDER

The Anatomy And Physiology Of The Shoulder Joint

One of the human body's most intricate and flexible joints is the shoulder joint. The humerus, which is the upper arm bone, the scapula, which is the shoulder blade, and the clavicle, which is the collarbone, make up this ball-and-socket joint. The ball-and-socket mechanism is formed by the humerus's head fitting into the glenoid, a shallow cavity in the scapula. Because of its broad range of motion, the shoulder can perform a variety of actions, including lifting, rotating, and swinging.

Multiple key components stabilize the shoulder joint. The glenoid's labrum, a ring of cartilage surrounding it, aids in deepening the socket and giving the humeral head a more snug fit. Further support is provided by the fibrous tissue envelope that encloses the joint, known as the joint capsule. Ligaments that connect bones and prevent excessive movement that can cause dislocation, such as the glenohumeral and coracohumeral ligaments, also play a role.

The Rotator Cuff Muscles' Function

Four muscles and the tendons that go with them make up the rotator cuff, which is essential to shoulder function. The teres minor, subscapularis, infraspinatus, and supraspinatus are these muscles. They form a cuff around the joint by attaching to the head of the humerus after emerging from the scapula.

Every rotator cuff muscle has a distinct purpose. The arm can be raised away from the body with the help of the supraspinatus. The subscapularis aids in internal rotation of the shoulder, whilst the infraspinatus and teres minor are in charge of outward rotation. These muscles cooperate to stabilize the shoulder joint, guaranteeing that the humerus' head remains securely positioned inside the glenoid cavity as the arm is moved.

The Value Of Stability In The Shoulders

The upper limb cannot function well without shoulder stability. A mix of passive components (labrum, ligaments, and bones) and active structures (muscles, especially the rotator cuff) provide stability. The shoulder joint would be vulnerable to dislocations and subluxations, in which the humerus's head partially or falls out of the glenoid cavity, in the absence of sufficient support.

It is possible to perform precise and controlled movements by preserving shoulder stability. It is especially crucial for tasks that require lifting, pushing, or tugging—many of which are seen in sports and everyday activities. For example, to perform at their peak, athletes like tennis players or baseball pitchers rely largely on a solid shoulder. In addition to lowering the chance of injury, a secure shoulder joint promotes long-term joint health.

Recognizing The Range Of Motion In The Shoulders

One of the most well-known physical attributes of the shoulder joint is its wide range of motion, encompassing flexion, extension, abduction, adduction, and rotation. The arm's ability to move in almost all directions is mainly attributable to the joint's ball-and-socket construction.

Arm extension is the movement of the arm backward, and arm flexion is the elevation of the arm forward. Raising the arm away from the midline of the body is known as abduction, and bringing it back towards the body is known as adduction.

An arm can rotate either internally, turning it inside, or externally, turning it outward. These motions are necessary for carrying out daily tasks including reaching for items, getting dressed, and engaging in physical activity or sports.

Sustaining the entire range of mobility in the shoulder is essential for both quality of life and functional independence. Many ailments, such as rotator cuff tears, frozen shoulder, or arthritis, can cause restricted shoulder movement and greatly impair a person's capacity to carry out daily duties.

Typical Injuries To The Shoulders

Shoulder injuries are common and can be caused by either long-term misuse or abrupt trauma. Rotator cuff tears, shoulder impingement, dislocations, and labral tears are a few of the most typical shoulder injuries.

Rotator cuff tears can result from progressive wear and tear or from an abrupt accident like lifting a heavy weight. Pain, weakness, and restricted range of motion are common symptoms. When the rotator cuff tendons are pinched during arm motions, it results in shoulder impingement, which causes discomfort and irritation.

Dislocations happen when the humeral head is pushed out of the glenoid cavity, frequently by a blow or a fall. For the joint to be relocated and additional damage to be avoided, this injury requires emergency medical intervention. Pain and instability can be caused by labral tears, which affect the cartilage around the shoulder socket and may arise from trauma or repetitive motions.

It is essential to comprehend these injuries and their mechanisms to avoid, detect, and treat them effectively. To reduce the chance of shoulder injuries and preserve ideal shoulder health, proper training, strengthening exercises, and ergonomic measures can be implemented.

CHAPTER TWO

ROTATOR CUFF TEARS: TYPES

Tears Of Partial Vs. Full Thickness

Partial and full-thickness tears are the two main classifications for rotator cuff tears. A partial tear occurs when some of the tendon is damaged but not all of it; as a result, the tendon is frayed but not destroyed.

Although there may still be some shoulder movement possible, these tears frequently result in pain and weakening in the shoulder. Because partial rips can present with variable degrees of discomfort and functional impairment, diagnosing them can be challenging at times.

On the other hand, a full-thickness rip, sometimes referred to as a complete tear, occurs when the tendon splits into two or separates from the bone. This kind of rupture causes severe shoulder weakness and loss of function, which frequently makes it challenging to raise the arm or carry out daily tasks. To restore shoulder function, full-thickness tears are usually more severe and frequently need surgical intervention.

Acute versus Prolonged Tears

Acute or chronic rotator cuff injuries can also be categorized according to when they first occur. An abrupt, violent incident, like lifting a large object, landing on an outstretched arm, or taking a direct hit to the shoulder, is usually the cause of acute tears. These tears frequently cause rapid loss of shoulder function and acute discomfort. Younger people and athletes who participate in high-impact activities are more likely to sustain acute tears.

On the other hand, chronic tears appear gradually over time as a result of tendon degeneration, wear and tear, or repetitive tension. Older persons and those whose jobs or hobbies include repetitive shoulder movements are more likely to have them. Although they might not hurt right away, chronic rips can result in gradual shoulder weakening, restricted range of motion, and ongoing discomfort. Treatment and recovery plans might be influenced by knowing whether a tear is acute or chronic.

Where And How Much Weeping There Is

The location and degree of a rotator cuff tear play a crucial role in dictating the best course of action for treatment.

Several rotator cuff tendons, including the infraspinatus, teres minor, and subscapularis tendons, can sustain tears. The supraspinatus tendon sustains tears the most frequently. The particular tendon that is torn can affect the symptoms that are felt as well as the functional restrictions that the tear imposes.

The magnitude of the tear is frequently used to determine severity. Conservative therapies, such as physical therapy, may be used to repair small tears (less than 1 cm), which can occasionally result in moderate symptoms. Large tears (3-5 cm) and medium tears (1-3 cm) typically cause more serious impairment and may need to be repaired surgically or with a combination of therapy.

Large tears (more than 5 cm) usually involve several tendons and pose a challenging clinical situation.

Surgical intervention is typically required to relieve discomfort and restore function.

Factors Affecting The Formation Of Tears

Rotator cuff tears can occur due to several reasons. Age plays a major role since rotator cuff tendons atrophy and degrade with age, making older people more prone to tears.

Both industrial and recreational repetitive overhead actions can overstress the rotator cuff, causing microtrauma and ultimately rupture.

A bad posture can also affect shoulder mechanics and put more strain on the rotator cuff tendons, among other issues.

Given that certain people are born with a propensity for poorer connective tissues, genetic predisposition might be involved. Furthermore, several illnesses, including diabetes and hypercholesterolemia, can harm tendons and promote the formation of tears.

Both controlling and avoiding rotator cuff injuries can be made easier by being aware of these risk factors.

Diagnostic Imaging Methods

Precise identification of rotator cuff injuries is necessary for efficient treatment planning, and imaging methods are vital to this procedure.

An X-ray is usually part of the first evaluation process to rule out abnormalities of the bones and identify any associated disorders that may be contributing to the shoulder pain, such as arthritis or bone spurs.

When it comes to identifying rotator cuff tears, magnetic resonance imaging (MRI) is the gold standard.

With the ability to precisely visualize the rotator cuff tendons, the amount of the tear, and any concomitant muscle atrophy, magnetic resonance imaging (MRI) offers detailed images of both soft tissues and bones.

MRI can also be used to evaluate the involvement of other shoulder components and distinguish between partial and full-thickness rips.

Another useful imaging modality is ultrasound, particularly for dynamic assessment. It makes it possible to see the rotator cuff tendons in real-time while the shoulder rotates, which is very helpful for locating partial tears and directing treatments like cortisone injections. Ultrasound is more affordable and easily accessible than MRI, although being less detailed.

Arthroscopy is a minimally invasive surgical procedure that can be utilized for both diagnosis and treatment in certain situations.

A tiny camera is introduced into the shoulder joint during arthroscopy to provide a clear image of the rotator cuff tendons and enable prompt surgery if needed. When diagnosing complex tears that are challenging to assess with non-invasive imaging, this method is quite helpful.

CHAPTER THREE

RISK ELEMENTS AND ACTIONS

Increasing Age And Degenerative Modifications

Our bodies experience a variety of degenerative changes as we age, and the rotator cuff is especially vulnerable to this inevitable wear and tear.

The tendons in the rotator cuff might lose suppleness and strength, rendering them more prone to injury. People over 40 usually experience the onset of degenerative changes, which intensify with age.

These alterations may consist of microtear formation, tendon thinning, and tendon calcification. These changes lessen the tendon's capacity to tolerate tension, which raises the risk of rupture from even small strains or activities. Regular check-ups and early treatments can help manage these changes effectively.

Overindulgence And Repetitive Motions

The rotator cuff muscles are responsible for supporting the shoulder joint and facilitating a wide variety of movements. Overuse injuries can result from activities like painting, swimming, or tennis that require repetitive shoulder motions. Microtraumas to the tendons brought on by overuse can compound over time to cause serious harm.

Individuals who work in jobs or participate in sports that need repeated overhead motions are especially vulnerable. Overuse injuries can be considerably decreased by using the right techniques, taking regular pauses, and cross-training to distribute physical stress across different muscle groups.

Shoulder Accidents And Traumas

Acute trauma can result in acute damage to the rotator cuff from events like falls, accidents, or abrupt jerks. These occurrences may result in partial or total tendon tears, which are frequently accompanied by excruciating pain and shoulder dysfunction.

Although they are more common in younger, active people, traumatizing injuries can also happen to elderly folks, particularly those who already have degenerative abnormalities in their bodies.

It's critical to keep up a healthy physical condition, participate in activities responsibly, and wear protective gear as needed to reduce the danger.

Getting medical help as soon as possible after an injury will help to improve recovery results and stop more difficulties.

Techniques For Preventing Injuries

Combining flexibility training, strengthening exercises, and ergonomic changes can help prevent rotator cuff problems.

To maintain the shoulder joint and prevent injuries, it can be helpful to strengthen the surrounding stabilizers and the rotator cuff.

It's good to perform exercises like internal and external rotations, lateral lifts, and shoulder presses.

Stretching exercises are part of a flexibility training program that helps preserve a range of motion and minimize stiffness.

Using supportive chairs and avoiding repetitive overhead motions are two examples of ergonomic changes that can be made at work and during daily activities to help prevent accidents.

Lifestyle Changes For The Health Of The Shoulders

Maintaining the health of your shoulder and avoiding rotator cuff problems need you to have a healthy lifestyle.

Tendon health can be supported and inflammation can be decreased with a balanced diet full of foods high in anti-inflammatory nutrients such as fruits, vegetables, and omega-3 fatty acids.

Frequent exercise, such as strength training and aerobic activities, helps to maintain the general flexibility and strength of the body.

Furthermore, abstaining from alcohol and smoking is essential because these behaviors can reduce blood supply to the tendons and impede their ability to renew and mend.

The general health of the musculoskeletal system, including the rotator cuff, is also influenced by getting enough sleep and practicing mindfulness to manage stress.

CHAPTER FOUR

DIAGNOSIS AND ASSESSMENT

Medical Professionals' Clinical Evaluation

Upon diagnosing a rotator cuff tear, medical professionals begin with a comprehensive clinical evaluation. Compiling a thorough medical history and comprehending the patient's symptoms—including the beginning, course, and severity of shoulder pain—are important steps in this procedure. Doctors inquire about any recent injuries, activities that worsen the pain, and therapies that have been tried in the past. The purpose of the evaluation is to identify any patterns that might point to a rotator cuff injury.

In addition, medical professionals assess the patient's general health, taking into account variables that may affect the risk of a rotator cuff rupture, such as age, occupation, and degree of physical activity. They might ask about diabetes or arthritis, for example, as these disorders can also have an impact on shoulder health. Clinicians can have a better understanding of the shoulder pain's context and possible causes by assembling this thorough history.

Imaging Studies: Mris, Ultrasounds, And X-Rays

Imaging tests are essential for the diagnosis of rotator cuff injuries because they provide visual information that physical investigations cannot.

Usually, X-rays are the initial imaging method employed. They can't see soft tissues like the rotator cuff directly, but they can help rule out other diseases like fractures or bone spurs that could be causing shoulder pain. A clear picture of the bone structure can be obtained via X-rays, which can also reveal indications of arthritis or other abnormalities of the bone that may impact the shoulder joint.

When it comes to identifying rotator cuff tears, magnetic resonance imaging (MRI) is the gold standard. A magnetic resonance imaging (MRI) scan can precisely identify tears, determine the extent of damage, and assess the state of surrounding tissues such as muscles and tendons by providing detailed images of both soft tissue and bone. MRIs are very helpful in planning surgical procedures when needed since they give a clear picture of the anatomy of the shoulder.

Another useful technology is ultrasound, particularly considering how affordable and convenient it is. It enables dynamic examination, which enables medical professionals to watch the rotator cuff move.

This is useful for spotting tears that would not be apparent in still pictures. Additionally, ultrasound can be used to guide some therapeutic injections.

Methods Of Physical Examination

Healthcare professionals employ particular approaches to evaluate the shoulder's function and identify the cause of pain during the physical examination. These methods aid in assessing the shoulder joint's range of motion, muscular strength, and existence of any unusual movements or noises.

To diagnose impingement, a disorder frequently linked to rotator cuff injuries, two popular tests are the Neer Impingement Test and the Hawkins-Kennedy Test.

In these tests, the patient's arm is moved in predetermined directions by the examiner to assess if it causes pain, which would indicate impingement.

The goal of the Drop Arm Test and Supraspinatus Test is to identify rotator cuff muscle weakness.

In the Drop Arm Test, the patient carefully lowers their arm from an elevated position; a tear is suggested if the patient is unable to regulate this movement.

The supraspinatus muscle, a crucial component of the rotator cuff, is tested for strength and discomfort using the empty can test.

Differential Shoulder Pain Diagnosis

To differentiate rotator cuff tears from other diseases that cause shoulder pain, differential diagnosis is crucial.

The symptoms of a rotator cuff rupture can be mimicked by ailments like bursitis, adhesive capsulitis, frozen shoulder, and shoulder impingement syndrome.

Healthcare professionals take into account the unique aspects of every ailment to correctly differentiate.

For instance, rotator cuff tears frequently cause discomfort and weakness during particular movements, whereas a frozen shoulder usually manifests as a severe restriction in both active and passive ranges of motion.

Diagnostic complications can arise from conditions such as cervical radiculopathy that also cause pain that is referred to the shoulder. It may be essential to perform a comprehensive evaluation that includes nerve conduction investigations or electromyography to rule out these other diseases.

The Value Of Extensive Analysis

Accurately identifying a rotator cuff tear requires a thorough assessment. A thorough evaluation guarantees that the right diagnosis is obtained because of the intricacy of the shoulder joint and the variety of illnesses that might produce symptoms that are similar to one another.

This all-inclusive method involves obtaining a complete medical history, performing a comprehensive physical examination, and using the right imaging studies.

The cornerstone of any successful treatment is a precise diagnosis. It enables medical professionals to customize interventions based on the unique requirements of the patient, ranging from conservative management—such as physical therapy and medication—to surgical repair in more serious situations. Ensuring a holistic approach to patient care, a thorough evaluation also assists in detecting any coexisting illnesses that may influence treatment outcomes.

CHAPTER FIVE

SELECTIVE NON-SURGICAL ROTATOR CUFF TEAR TREATMENT OPTIONS

Elevation, Compression, Ice, Rest (RICE)

A common first therapy for many soft tissue injuries, including rotator cuff tears, is the RICE approach.

Resting entails refraining from activities that aggravate shoulder discomfort as the first stage.

This stops more harm from happening and lets the healing process start. You must avoid overhead movements and heavy lifting at this time.

Using ice helps numb the discomfort and minimize inflammation. For the first 48 hours following the injury, apply an ice pack wrapped in a cloth to the shoulder for 15 to 20 minutes every few hours. To relieve pain and edema, repeat this procedure multiple times daily.

Using an elastic bandage to compress the damaged region might help reduce swelling and give it extra support. But be careful not to compress too tightly to impede blood flow.

Maintaining the shoulder elevated—ideally above the level of the heart—entails elevation. Allowing fluids to drain away from the injured site, can assist minimize swelling. Use pillows to elevate your shoulder while you're sleeping.

Rehabilitation And Physical Therapy

An essential part of the non-surgical management of rotator cuff injuries is physical therapy. The goal of a customized physical therapy program is to rebuild shoulder function, strength, and flexibility. First, mild range-of-motion exercises are taught to preserve joint suppleness and avoid stiffness.

Strengthening activities are added as the recovery process advances. These exercises work the rotator cuff and shoulder blade muscles, which support and stabilize the shoulder joint. To guarantee correct form and prevent additional injury, it is imperative to carry out these exercises under the supervision of a physical therapist.

An additional component of rehabilitation is functional training. Progressively restoring the shoulder to regular usage, entails exercises and activities that mirror everyday tasks.

Maintaining the recommended physical treatment routine with consistency is essential for both a speedy recovery and the avoidance of further injuries.

Pain And Inflammation Medicines

An important part of managing rotator cuff injuries is controlling discomfort and inflammation.

Pain and swelling can be effectively reduced by over-the-counter nonsteroidal anti-inflammatory medicines (NSAIDs), such as naproxen and ibuprofen.

These drugs function by preventing the body from producing chemicals that lead to inflammation.

In certain situations, stronger prescription drugs might be required. These may consist of stronger NSAIDs or other painkillers.

Utilizing these drugs by a doctor's instructions is crucial to preventing any negative effects and drug interactions.

Acetaminophen, which lacks anti-inflammatory qualities, can be a viable substitute for NSAIDs in cases where a patient is unable to take them for pain management. Before beginning a new pharmaceutical regimen, always get medical advice.

Injections Of Corticosteroids

Severe pain and inflammation brought on by rotator cuff injuries can be significantly reduced by corticosteroid injections.

A corticosteroid drug is injected directly into the shoulder joint or the surrounding tissue during these injections.

The objective is to lessen pain and inflammation so that physical therapy and rehabilitation exercises become more manageable.

Corticosteroid injections can have a range of effects; some people feel better right once, while others may take a few days to see results.

It's crucial to remember that, even though these injections can be quite successful, their use is usually restricted to a few sessions annually due to possible adverse effects such as tendon weakness and an elevated risk of infection.

Based on the extent of the tear and the patient's reaction to previous treatments, a medical practitioner will decide on the best time and frequency of corticosteroid injections.

Treatment With Platelet-Rich Plasma (PRP)

To treat rotator cuff tears, a new treatment option called platelet-rich plasma (PRP) therapy harnesses the body's natural healing processes. A tiny amount of the patient's blood is drawn for PRP, which is then processed to concentrate the platelets and injected straight into the site of injury.

Growth factors found in platelets aid in tissue regeneration and repair. PRP therapy tries to decrease pain and hasten healing by concentrating these growth factors and administering them to the site of injury.

Because PRP therapy uses the patient's blood, there is less chance of allergic reactions or disease transmission, making it a relatively low-risk procedure.

PRP treatment, however, has a variable efficacy and might not be appropriate for all rotator cuff tears.

Before choosing this course of treatment, it is imperative to go over the possible advantages and disadvantages of a healthcare professional.

The best results are frequently obtained by combining the many non-surgical treatments for rotator cuff injuries, each of which offers a unique strategy. Effective recovery requires working with a healthcare provider to create a customized treatment plan.

CHAPTER SIX

SURGICAL ASSISTANCE

Reasons To Operate

When non-surgical therapies for rotator cuff injuries are ineffective, surgery is usually taken into consideration.

Surgery may be indicated if there is ongoing discomfort, particularly if it keeps you from sleeping or engaging in everyday activities, you have severe shoulder weakness, or you are unable to lift your arm.

Additionally, surgery can be required if the patient has a large tear, a tear brought on by a recent injury, or if they are a laborer or athlete who uses their shoulder frequently for work. Surgery may also be required for chronic tears that get worse over time or that don't get better with physical therapy.

Surgical Procedure Types

There are various surgical treatments for healing a rotator cuff tear, each suited to the individual type of damage.

Arthroscopic mend: This minimally invasive surgery involves small incisions through which a camera and specialized equipment are placed to visualize and mend the tear.

It is often favored due to its less intrusive nature, resulting in speedier recovery times.

Open Repair: In this more traditional method, a wider incision is made over the shoulder to enable direct access to the damaged tendon. This procedure is often utilized for larger or more difficult tears and allows for thorough mending.

Mini-Open Repair: This procedure combines arthroscopic and open surgery methods. Initially, arthroscopy is utilized to assess and partially treat the injury.

Then, a minor incision is made to complete the surgery. The goal of this strategy is to weigh the advantages of open and arthroscopic surgery.

Tendon Transfer: When a rotator cuff rupture cannot be repaired, a damaged tendon from another area of the body is used to replace it. For extensive tears, this is usually seen as a salvage surgery.

Shoulder Replacement: A shoulder replacement may be required in certain circumstances, especially if there is also severe arthritis. This entails using artificial elements to replace the shoulder's injured sections.

Open Vs Arthroscopic Surgery

The location and size of the tear, the patient's condition, and the surgeon's experience all play a role in choosing between arthroscopic and open surgery.

Because arthroscopic surgery is minimally invasive and produces smaller incisions, less discomfort, and quicker recovery times, it is frequently chosen.

It makes it possible to see the shoulder joint in great detail and to precisely heal the tear with the least amount of tissue disruption. After arthroscopic surgery, patients usually recover more quickly and resume their regular activities sooner.

Open surgery is a superior alternative for severe or complex tears that need direct visibility and substantial repair, even if it is more intrusive. With this technique, surgeons can simultaneously treat additional shoulder issues and carry out more complex repairs.

In contrast to arthroscopic surgery, open surgery typically entails greater postoperative pain and longer recovery periods.

The exact details of the tear as well as the patient's requirements and general state of health ultimately determine whether arthroscopic or open surgery is preferable.

Recovery After Surgery

A vital component of the healing process after rotator cuff surgery is rehabilitation. Immobilization is usually the first step in the process so that the repaired tendon can recover.

To prevent damage to the repair and limit shoulder movement, a sling must be worn for a few weeks.

Phase 1: Immobilization and Passive Motion: Under the supervision of a physical therapist, passive motion exercises are started in the initial weeks following surgery.

These exercises include the therapist moving the patient's arm to maintain flexibility without the patient actively activating their muscles.

Phase 2: Active Motion: Patients progressively start active motion exercises following the initial phase of recuperation.

To improve shoulder function, this phase focuses on restoring range of motion and incorporates mild stretching and strengthening activities.

Phase 3: Strengthening: The goal of the rehabilitation program is to strengthen the shoulder muscles as the healing process advances. To increase stability and repair strength, resistance workouts are introduced. To guarantee a complete recovery and avoid further injuries, this stage is essential.

Phase 4: Functional Training: This last stage entails functional training customized to the patient's activities or way of life. Exercises aimed at enhancing the shoulder's capacity to carry out regular duties, occupational activities, or sports-specific motions fall under this category.

Following the therapy program exactly is necessary for a full recovery. Consistent follow-ups with the surgeon and physical therapist guarantee appropriate healing and optimal function of the shoulder.

Possible Dangers And Issues

Although rotator cuff surgery is usually risk-free, there are certain hazards involved. One of the possible outcomes is infection, which could call for more surgery or medication. Additionally, patients may develop shoulder stiffness or loss of motion, which may call for further physical therapy or, in extreme circumstances, surgery.

Another concern is nerve injury, which can result in loss of function, weakness, or numbness in the arm or shoulder. A rare but dangerous post-operative complication that can happen is blood clots.

Additionally, if the patient returns to demanding activities too soon or if the initial rupture is big, there is a chance that the tendon will rip again. There are situations where the repaired tendon does not fully heal, leaving the patient with ongoing pain or disability.

After rotator cuff surgery, many patients report considerable improvements in pain and function, despite these concerns. To reduce difficulties and achieve a good result, a comprehensive preoperative examination, expert surgical technique, and attention to postoperative rehabilitation protocols are essential.

CHAPTER SEVEN

CARE AFTER POSTOPERATION AND REHABILITATION

Postoperative Rehabilitation's Significance

For those who have had rotator cuff tear surgery, postoperative therapy is an essential part of their recovery. Proper rehabilitation guarantees maximum recovery, restores strength and function, and lowers the risk of problems while surgery treats the physical damage to the rotator cuff. It serves as a sort of transition between surgery and getting back to your regular routines.

Regaining range of motion (ROM) in the shoulder joint is one of the main objectives of postoperative therapy. Movement may be restricted after surgery if scar tissue develops around the treated tendons. Exercises that increase the range of motion assist in gradually removing this scar tissue, restoring a greater range of motion to the shoulder. Usually, these activities begin slowly and increase in difficulty as the patient heals.

Exercises For Range Of Motion

The goal of range-of-motion exercises is to progressively improve the shoulder joint's flexibility and mobility. Pendulum swings, passive stretches, and aided range-of-motion exercises with the help of a physical therapist or with the use of instruments like pulleys are a few examples of these activities. To guarantee these exercises are done correctly and securely, it's crucial to carry them out under the supervision of a healthcare provider.

Range-of-motion exercises during the early phases of rehabilitation emphasize light motions to avoid putting too much stress on the healing tissues.

You can progressively increase the range and intensity of these workouts as your shoulder heals. Since consistency is essential to getting the best outcomes, patients are frequently advised to incorporate these exercises into their regular rehabilitation regimen.

Programs For Strengthening And Conditioning

After achieving a sufficient range of motion, the emphasis switches to building up the muscles that surround the shoulder joint. Exercises for strengthening the muscles aid in the reconstruction of any weaker muscles brought on by the accident or surgery. Along with other shoulder-supporting and -stabilizing muscles including the deltoids and scapular stabilizers, the rotator cuff muscles are the focus of these exercises.

Programs for conditioning and strength training are customized for each person based on their unique requirements and objectives. Resistance training with weights, resistance bands, or bodyweight exercises are examples of exercises. These exercises improve total functional capacity and help develop shoulder muscle strength and endurance by gradually increasing resistance and intensity.

Returning To Activities Gradually

Patients can progressively resume their regular activities as their strength, flexibility, and function improve during rehabilitation. To avoid re-injury, it's crucial to go cautiously and refrain from exerting yourself. Advice on when to resume sports, heavy lifting, or repetitive overhead motions can be obtained from physical therapists or other medical professionals.

Patients may continue with a modified rehabilitation regimen to maintain progress and avoid setbacks during the return to activities phase. This could entail regular strength and flexibility training in addition to instruction on good body mechanics and techniques for preventing injuries.

Keeping An Eye Out For Complications Or Recurrence

Monitoring must continue even after rehabilitation is complete and normal activities are resumed to identify any complications or recurrences. This could involve routine check-ups with medical professionals, imaging tests like MRI scans, and continuing self-evaluations for symptoms like pain, weakness, or restricted range of motion.

Timely treatment and damage prevention can be achieved by detecting recurrences or problems early on and taking appropriate action.

To guarantee the best possible results and long-term shoulder health, patients are advised to notify their healthcare practitioner of any concerns or changes in their symptoms as soon as possible.

CHAPTER EIGHT

CHANGES IN LIFESTYLE AND LONG-TERM MANAGEMENT

Long-term management and prevention of rotator cuff injuries depend heavily on lifestyle changes. These modifications cover a wide range of day-to-day activities, such as diet, exercise, ergonomics, and mental health procedures. People can improve their general health and reduce the chance of further rotator cuff injuries by putting these changes into practice.

Ergonomic Adjustments To Stop Recurrence

Ergonomic modifications entail streamlining everyday tasks and the workspace to lessen shoulder strain and stop rotator cuff tears from happening again. This entails utilizing ergonomic devices like supporting chairs and keyboards, altering workstation and chair heights to guarantee good posture, and avoiding repetitive motions that place unnecessary strain on the shoulder joint. Additionally, rotator cuff protection during daily work can be achieved by changing lifting techniques to engage the core muscles and distribute weight uniformly.

Nutrition And Hydration's Role

To promote the healing process and preserve general shoulder health, nutrition is essential. Consuming a diet high in fruits, vegetables, lean meats, and omega-3 fatty acids can supply vital nutrients for reducing inflammation and repairing tissue. Drinking enough water is crucial for maintaining joint lubrication and preventing cramping caused by dehydration in the muscles. Including these eating practices into everyday life can help you recover from rotator cuff injuries as best you can and manage them over the long run.

The Value Of Frequent Exercise

Frequent exercise is crucial for increasing the range of motion, flexibility, and strength in the muscles that surround the shoulder joint. Exercises that target the rotator cuff, like internal and external rotations, can aid in the restoration of stability and strength in the injured area.

Furthermore, adding cardiovascular and general strength training to a schedule can improve overall fitness and maintain joint health.

To prevent aggravating the injury, it's imperative to begin cautiously and increase intensity gradually. For individualized exercise recommendations, speak with a physical therapist or healthcare professional.

Stress Reduction And Mental Health

Long-term care for rotator cuff tears must include both stress management and upholding mental wellness. Mobility restrictions and chronic pain can hurt mental health, increasing the risk of anxiety, sadness, and a lower standard of living.

Deep breathing, mindfulness, and meditation are examples of relaxation practices that can be used to reduce stress and foster tranquility. In addition, getting help from loved ones, friends, or a mental health professional can offer coping mechanisms and emotional support while going through the healing process.

Long-Term Care Follow-Up With Medical Professionals

It is crucial to schedule routine follow-up appointments with medical professionals to track development, treat any residual symptoms, and modify treatment regimens as necessary. This can entail routine evaluations of shoulder function, range of motion, and strength by a primary care physician, physical therapist, or orthopedic specialist. To assess the healing process and find any underlying problems, imaging procedures like MRIs and X-rays may be advised. Having open lines of contact with medical professionals guarantees comprehensive care and empowers patients to decide on their course of treatment and rehabilitation objectives.

CHAPTER NINE

COMMON QUESTIONS AND ANSWERS

A rotator cuff injury may give rise to several queries and worries. Knowing these often-asked questions might help people feel less anxious and point them in the direction of the right care and rehabilitation techniques.

Can Tears In The Rotator Cuff Heal On Their Own?

The severity of rotator cuff injuries varies, and while some may recover with conservative measures, others might need surgery. Small tears or strains may heal with rest, ice, and physical therapy exercises designed to increase flexibility and strengthen the surrounding muscles. Larger tears, on the other hand, or those that result in severe discomfort and dysfunction frequently call for medical intervention. To ascertain the optimal course of action for each unique case, speaking with a healthcare professional is essential.

What Are Surgical Intervention Success Rates?

Good results can be obtained with surgery for rotator cuff injuries, especially if the procedure is carried out by a skilled surgeon and is followed by rigorous rehabilitation. Success rates are influenced by several variables, including the location and size of the tear, the general health of the patient, and compliance with postoperative care instructions. After surgery, the majority of patients typically see notable improvements in their general quality of life, pain reduction, and functional restoration. To make well-informed judgments regarding treatment alternatives, it is imperative to consult a healthcare expert about expectations and potential hazards.

How Much Time Does Recovery Take?

The length of time it takes for patients to recover from rotator cuff tears varies and is influenced by several variables, including the degree of the tear, the treatment plan selected, and the patient's capacity for healing. When surgery is necessary, the shoulder is usually immobilized for a while before gradually regaining strength, range of motion, and flexibility with rehabilitation activities. A full recovery could take many months, with the first few weeks being devoted to pain relief and repair protection, then gradually increasing the intensity of workouts to reestablish shoulder function. A good recovery depends on following the recommendations of medical specialists and adhering to the rehabilitation regimen as prescribed.

After Treatment, Will My Whole Range Of Motion Return?

Following rotator cuff tear therapy, regaining full range of motion is contingent upon several circumstances, such as the extent of the tear, the efficacy of the selected course of treatment, and the rehabilitation progress of each patient. Some people may fully recover their shoulder function, while others may still have lingering restrictions, especially if they have large tears or underlying degenerative diseases. Physical therapy is essential for maximizing range of motion since it helps to release tight muscles, loosen up stiff joints, and enhance shoulder mechanics in general. Achieving functional goals can be increased with consistent participation in recommended workouts and continued discussion with healthcare practitioners.

How Can I Avoid Shoulder Injuries In The Future?

A proactive strategy that emphasizes strengthening the muscles around the shoulder joint, increasing flexibility, and using the right body mechanics when engaging in daily activities and sports is necessary to prevent future shoulder injuries.

Exercises that strengthen the rotator cuff muscles, like scapular stabilization and external rotation, can improve shoulder stability and lower the chance of injury. Keeping a healthy weight, avoiding overhead motions repeatedly, and employing safe lifting techniques can all help reduce the chance of developing rotator cuff tears and other shoulder issues. To maintain total shoulder health and prevent injuries, regular participation in a well-rounded fitness program that incorporates both strength training and flexibility activities is recommended.

www.ingramcontent.com/pod-product-compliance
Lightning Source LLC
Chambersburg PA
CBHW071841210526
45479CB00001B/236